Elsie Antonieta Saavedra Alvarado
Carlos Julio Saavedra Alvarado
Maddelyn Teresa Cotto Aguilar

Intervention plan to prevent occupational hazards

Elsie Antonieta Saavedra Alvarado
Carlos Julio Saavedra Alvarado
Maddelyn Teresa Cotto Aguilar

Intervention plan to prevent occupational hazards

Hospital sterilization area

Imprint

Any brand names and product names mentioned in this book are subject to trademark, brand or patent protection and are trademarks or registered trademarks of their respective holders. The use of brand names, product names, common names, trade names, product descriptions etc. even without a particular marking in this work is in no way to be construed to mean that such names may be regarded as unrestricted in respect of trademark and brand protection legislation and could thus be used by anyone.

Cover image: www.ingimage.com

This book is a translation from the original published under ISBN 978-620-0-03340-6.

Publisher:
Sciencia Scripts
is a trademark of
Dodo Books Indian Ocean Ltd. and OmniScriptum S.R.L publishing group

120 High Road, East Finchley, London, N2 9ED, United Kingdom
Str. Armeneasca 28/1, office 1, Chisinau MD-2012, Republic of Moldova, Europe
Managing Directors: Ieva Konstantinova, Victoria Ursu
info@omniscriptum.com

Printed at: see last page
ISBN: 978-620-2-77968-5

INTERVENTION PLAN TO PREVENT OCCUPATIONAL RISK IN THE STERILISATION AREA.

AUTHORS:

LIC. SAAVEDRA ALVARADO ELSIE ANTONIETA, MGS. SAAVEDRA ALVARADO CARLOS JULIO, MGS.
LIC. COTTO AGUILAR MADDELYN TERESA, MGS.

DEDICATION

We dedicate this research to the LORD GOD Almighty and to our FATHERS AND BROTHERS.
To JEHOVAH GOD Almighty because he has been with us every step we take, taking care of us and giving us strength to continue, to my PARENTS AND BROTHERS, who throughout our lives have watched over our welfare and training being the support at all times. They have placed their complete trust in every challenge we have faced, never doubting our intelligence and capacity for a single moment.
That is why we are what we are now.
Authors

THANK YOU

To JEHOVAH GOD Almighty for being the transcendental objective of our path who allowed us to go forward fighting in search of our progress, with humility, simplicity and dedication in order to achieve each objective.
To my PARENTS and BROTHERS for their sharpness and unconditional support to complete this stage of my professional life.
Authors

TABLE OF CONTENTS

EXECUTIVE SUMMARY

The primordial objective of the present investigative work is the proposal of a Plan of Intervention to avoid the labor risk in the sterilization area in The General Hospital   Dr. Liborio Panchana Sotomayor, Canton Santa Elena, and County Santa Elena.

Before executing the design of the outlined proposal, an analysis of the components was made that conform the strategies to avoid the labor risks, to have theoretical bases and to be able to fulfill to cabal dad the proposed objective.

The primordial source of information is the interviews that were carried out to those involved with the process like they are; Nurses who manifested the necessity to improve and to avoid the labor risks, also the carried out surveys that they were of maximum it contributes, because they contributed to verify the idea to defend of the present work.

The progress of this investigation is based bibliographically by means of scientifically proven theories that guided the structure of the intervention plan to avoid the labor risk in the sterilization area.

Lately the proposal was constituted in base of the design of an intervention plan that is based on three elements, which will allow: 1. I design and systematizing of a training plan, 2. Plan of labor health and prevention of risks, 3. Chronogram of socialization of the training in risks and measures of labor prevention.

Key words*: plan, risks, administration, indicators, health, factors.*

INTRODUCTION

Background to Research.

The objective of occupational risks in the sterilisation area is to identify the risks that may occur with health personnel, to determine the negative effects caused by these risks, to draw up a plan of measures aimed at preventing them, and also to serve as a tool to unify prevention criteria.

The vast majority of accidents at work are avoidable, especially the serious and fatal ones; accidents at work are not the consequence of a biblical curse or an unavoidable tribute of work, accidents are the result of the consequence of the lack of preventive practices that in their nature are knowable and applicable, it is precisely the lack of implementation of such measures, the causes of accidents and other damage to the health of workers, according to the research conducted by Dra. María de Lourdes Velasco at the Carlos Andrade Marín Hospital in the city of Quito in 2018. (Velasco, 2018)

The occupational risks that exist in the area of sterilisation include all physical, mechanical, biological and preferably chemical procedures used to destroy pathogenic germs in which critical and semi-critical manoeuvres are carried out, as the personnel run the risk of suffering intoxication, burns, pulmonary problems and visual fatigue, and the personnel who work in this area are not aware of the Manual of Standards and Procedures of the Ministry of Public Health, 2020. (Public Health, 2020)

In addition to the risks associated with the activity itself and independent of the type of sterilisation carried out, such as the handling of loads or repetitive movements, the different processes to achieve sterility entail a series of dangers inherent to the nature of the process itself, ranging from burns associated with high temperatures to the carcinogenic and mutagenic nature of some of chemical sterilising agents, according to Castro Sabio, Alfonso Psychologist. Unidad Periférica de Prevención de Riesgos Laborales/Servicio de Medicina Preventiva / Complejo Hospitalario Universitario Juan Canalejo, Spain 2017. (Castro, 2017)

For (NIOSH) Publication No. 2000-108 November 2007. "Occupational hazards in sterilisation; they can be acute and chronic infections, allergic and toxic reactions caused by biological agents and their derivatives, demonstrating the need to establish a Manual of Standards and Procedures on occupational hazards in the central sterilisation unit". (NIOSH, 2007)According to Martha Rodríguez González of the International Centre for Neurological Restoration (CIREN), Havana, Cuba (2015). The sterilisation centre in a health centre is considered the heart of the centre, since it is where almost all the materials used for critical and semi-critical manoeuvres in the clinical care of patients are stored, and which must undergo a cleaning, disinfection and sterilisation process; it is also responsible for storing and distributing the necessary medical-surgical material and for preparing the material for cures. Nowadays, due to the high scientific level reached, the performance of complex procedures is increasing, which requires medical devices with optimal quality (Rodriguez, 2015).

The problem statement.

In Spain, in the area of sterilisation, one of most relevant problems in terms of accidents at work and occupational diseases is undoubtedly misinformation. Information is fundamental, not as a finalist action, but as a means to further deepen the knowledge of the situations in our environment and specifically in the workplace, knowledge of working conditions. In the same way, if we take a sample among citizens as to which resources they value and believe to be a priority, the majority will answer health and information. (Patón, 2021).

In El Salvador, at the beginning of 2008, occupational accidents were legally regulated and currently there are few institutions that promote occupational health and safety such as: the Ministry of Labour and Social Security through the Department of Occupational Health, the Salvadoran Social Security Institute through the Department of Occupational Health and the Industrial Foundation for the Prevention of Occupational Risks (FIPRO), showing lack of socialisation of an Occupational Risk Protection Plan. in the sterilisation area of hospital units in Central American countries (Escuela de Ingenieria Biomédica, 2017).

In the city of Bogotá, in the Hospital Universitario San Ignacio, a highly complex health service provider, the risks to which workers are exposed are classified as Type II risk, according to the economic activity of health. The occupational accident indicators for 2008 show a total of 185 accidents, 93 of which were biological (50.2%) and 92 non-biological (49.8%), due to the absence of an occupational risk intervention plan in the establishment, especially in the sterilisation centre to prevent damage to the health of the workers. (Ignacio, 2020).

According to the Pan American Health Organisation in 2022, the occupational risks to which health workers are exposed are well documented and generally fall into the following six basic categories: biological or infectious risks, environmental risks, physical risks, chemical risks, mechanical risks and psychosocial risks, which should be socialised to all working in the sterilisation centres of each hospital unit in order to raise awareness and occupational accidents.

The World Health Organisation states that the cornerstone of biosafety practice is risk assessment. Although many tools exist to help assess the risk involved in a given procedure or experiment, the most important component is professional judgement. Risk assessments should be carried out by those with the best knowledge of the specific characteristics of the organisms to be worked on, the equipment and procedures to be used, with the aim of reducing potential risks in the workplace. (WHO, 2023).

In Ecuador, the Ministry of Public Health is responsible for regulating, monitoring and taking measures to protect human health from the risks and damage that may be caused by environmental conditions. Through Ministerial Agreement N° 001005 published in the Official Register N° 106 of 10 January 1997, the Regulations for the Appropriate Management of Infectious Waste Generated in Health Institutions in were issued, but the supervision of health units is not fully carried out. (MSP, 2022). In our Nation, in the Province of Cotopaxi, in General Hospital of Latacunga, in an investigation carried out progressively since 2009, multiple risk factors were observed in the workers who work in the sterilisation centre that can affect their well-being and integrity, being essential to offer quality services to the user, being necessary to establish and carry out an intervention plan for occupational risks in the sterilisation area to reduce the risks to which each personnel is subject. (Fierro, 2021).

Hospital establishments are framed within the economic activity of the services, and a variety of occupational hazards can be found there, including biological, chemical, physical and ergonomic risks, which can cause illness and death in their workers, and can be regulated by proposing an intervention plan to disseminate and promote the workers of the sterilisation centres as a management , since there is no plan to prevent occupational accidents in the institution. (Aguilar, 2021).

The Ministry of Public Health of Ecuador SINCE 2019, states that the sterilisation , which functionally, is responsible for providing clinical-sterilised materials, a support element for the prevention of hospital infections, where there is no plan to prevent occupational hazards in each sterilisation centre. In view of the above, it is necessary to monitor these activities in order to prevent occupational accidents among the personnel working in this area, promoting an intervention plan for occupational risks and training workers.

At national level, the work situation, the sum of human activity and technology, can cause environmental alterations that generate risk situations, which are defined as uncontrolled work situations, in which unforeseen phenomena can occur when planning the work process, such as errors, incidents, breakdowns, production defects, accidents at work and occupational diseases, it is necessary to draw up an Intervention Plan on occupational risks to intensify the teaching of personnel. health care providers about the risks involved and to avoid possible harm to personal integrity.

The General Hospital Dr. Liborio Panchana Sotomayor Liborio Panchana Sotomayor General Hospital is the most complex unit of the health services network in the Province of Santa Elena, governed by policies and regulations dictated by the Ministry of Public Health of Ecuador, based on the principles of solidarity, universality and equity, to provide comprehensive, ethical, up-to-date and specialised medical care, It should be noted that such training should be prioritised in areas of greatest occupational risk, such as the Sterilisation Centre, which has nine nursing assistants (it does not have nursing professionals), to guide the training and thus orient the staff on occupational hazards.

It is a second level hospital that attends to health problems of all medical specialties, it is a provincial reference unit, which promotes education, information, communication for the general community of the city and the province of Santa Elena, the sterilisation area is where there is the greatest occupational risk.

Its vision is to be a leading hospital in health care at a national level, with economic and administrative autonomy, framed in the legal principles of the Ministry of Public Health of Ecuador, with an organisational model within the Health System, providing comprehensive and specialised care. It seeks to achieve excellence in its services in order to satisfy and exceed the needs and expectations of its clients.

The occupational hazards that exist in the sterilisation area include all physical, mechanical, biological and preferably chemical procedures, which are used to destroy pathogenic germs in which critical manoeuvres are carried out (instruments or objects that are introduced directly into the bloodstream, e.g. surgical instruments, implants, etc.) and semi-critical manoeuvres (which come into contact with the patient's intact mucous membranes, e.g. endotracheal tubes, etc.), as the personnel are at risk of suffering from poisoning and contamination.(instruments or objects that are in contact with intact mucous membranes of the patient, e.g. surgical instruments, implants, etc.) and semi-critical (in contact with intact mucous membranes of the patient, e.g. endotracheal tubes), as the personnel are at risk of poisoning, burns, eye irritation, lung problems, eyestrain, falls, allergies, cuts, fires, constant handling of contaminated material, lighting, noise, equipment failure, heat, electric shocks, sterilising gases, lifting of heavy instrumental equipment.

The personnel working in this area do not have knowledge of the Manual of Standards, Procedures and Biosafety Measures because the administrative area has not paid attention to this area in order to have a highly trained and permanent staff, there are no signs to differentiate between contaminated and sterile areas, there is no frequent training for their knowledge, as they only work with auxiliary personnel and they do not have professional personnel in charge of them, where supervision is carried out to make decisions to avoid accidents at work in the sterilisation centre.

In the sterilisation area, it is necessary to determine the negative effects that these risks have on health, and an intervention plan should be drawn up to prevent them, as well as tools that should be adopted to the safety standards and recommendations so that the personnel can obtain the corresponding protections.

It is therefore necessary for the administrative area to identify the occupational risks in the sterilisation , which has a deficient and insufficient staff with inadequate procedures for carrying out its own tasks. The identification of occupational risks makes it possible to estimate the magnitude of those risks found in a specific work process and, based on these risks, to establish preventive measures with the aim of minimising or eliminating them, prevention planning is necessary, adapting the risk control measures to each work post, to each function that the worker carries out, and even to the physical and biological conditions of each person under the model of an intervention plan in the sterilisation area.

It is part of administrative management process to supervise and monitor quality indicators in order to analyse the existing dangers to avoid occupational risks to which the personnel working in the sterilisation area of the General Hospital Dr. Liborio Panchana Sotomayor are exposed, as there is no Occupational Risk Intervention Plan in place. At the managerial and administrative level, standards and protocols must be managed to solve "performance problems". In this sense, the original source of information is the performance evaluation that should be carried out periodically in the service, as well as the diagnostic studies of needs, aimed at identifying and determining which are feasible to solve through an intervention plan in the sterilisation area. It can be determined that knowledge is the most important element that a person possesses in order to develop the perception of risk necessary to protect health, a condition from which workers in the sterilisation area are not exempt, as they must specify and incorporate prevention measures into their daily practices in the different work positions, with the objective of preserving health and contributing to protecting the health of patients.

Formulation of the problem

How to avoid occupational accidents to health personnel working in the sterilisation area of the General Hospital Dr. Liborio Panchana, Cantón Santa Elena are exposed?

Delimitation of the problem

The good intentions to occupational accidents to which health personnel are exposed will help to ensure that 100% of them are trained, for which it is important to delimit the space and time of the object of study.
Spatial delimitation: This study was carried out in the General Hospital Dr. Liborio Pancha Sotomayor, Santa Elena canton. Province of Santa Elena.
Time frame: this research was carried out in the first half of the year 2024.

Object of the research and field of action.

The object of the research is framed within the framework of occupational health.
The field of action in the reduction of occupational risk in the sterilisation area.

Identification of the Line of Research.

The line of research for this research is: Health Services Management.
Objective general.

To design an intervention plan to avoid occupational risk in the sterilisation area of the General Hospital Dr. Liborio Panchana Sotomayor, Canton Santa Elena, Province of Santa Elena.

Objectives specific.

✓ Theoretical and scientific basis for an intervention plan to prevent accidents at work in the sterilisation area of the Dr. Liborio Panchana Sotomayor Hospital, Canton Santa Elena, Province of Santa Elena.
➢ To diagnose the occupational risk factors to which the staff working in the different areas of the sterilisation centre of the Dr. Liborio Panchana Sotomayor Hospital are exposed.
✓ Elaborate the elements of the intervention plan to avoid work-related accidents the sterilisation area of the Dr. Liborio Panchana Sotomayor Hospital, Canton Santa Elena, Province of Santa Elena.
✓ Validate the proposal through expert channels

Idea to Defender.

With the design of an Occupational Risk Intervention Plan to improve the quality of personnel, occupational accidents in the sterilisation area of the Dr. Liborio Panchana Sotomayor Hospital, Canton Santa Elena, Province of Santa Elena would be avoided.

Variables of the research.

Independent variable:Intervention Plan.
Dependent Variable:Decrease in occupational risk.

Justification of the theme.

The research project has the characteristics, technical and operational conditions that ensure the fulfilment of its goals and objectives.
In every health institution, the protection of human resources with regard to risks during their working day must be guaranteed as part of its management, depending on the area in which they work.
We can determine which occupational hazards are the dangers existing in our work task or in our own environment or workplace, which can cause accidents or any type of accidents that, in turn, are factors that can cause injuries, physical or psychological damage, trauma, etc.
Whereby risk is the likelihood of harm occurring as a result of exposure. Any characteristic of the work that may have a significant influence on the generation of risks to the safety and health of workers.
For this purpose, we will carry out a retrospective, cross-sectional study whose universe will be the nursing staff working in the sterilisation area.
With this background, we are considering carrying out a research project based on an intervention plan to prevent occupational hazards in the sterilisation area of the General Hospital Dr. Liborio Panchana Sotomayor, Santa Elena canton, Santa Elena province. Therefore, this study will respond to methodologies that will be used in the investigative context that will contribute to identifying the causes or factors that predominate in the problem posed.
In order to reduce occupational risk in the sterilisation area in the population under study. The aim is to seek strategies to prevent accidents at work under an intervention plan that will benefit the overall health of employees.

Research methodology to be used: technical methods and tools used in the research.

The aim of the research is to find out about national entities in charge of developing policies, standards and procedures for the prevention and control of accidents, risks and illnesses in the area of sterilisation. In addition, to get to know those entities that collaborate in the process of prevention of accidents and occupational illnesses by means of advice or consultancy.

The types of research to be carried out are:

The data collection was carried out using two methods

Bibliographic research. Books on planning, management, administration and safety in the sterilisation area; safety manuals and guides; articles published on the Internet; norms and standards promulgated by associations and organisations were consulted.

Interviews: Evaluative interviews (to obtain information) and structured interviews (following a procedure established beforehand by a survey, questionnaire or guide) will be carried out in the sterilisation area of the General Hospital Dr. Liborio Panchana Sotomayor.

Surveys: this was carried out among the personnel working in the sterilisation area in order to find out about occupational hazards.

The research methods to be used are:

Inductive-Deductive: Applied to generate a particular response to the problem and then generalise it to the authorities of the Dr. Liborio Panchana Sotomayor Hospital.

Analytical-synthetic: Applied to analyse information required to solve the problem and synthesised in the theoretical framework.

Theoretical contribution, practical significance and scientific novelty.

To ensure that the Sterilisation area's information management process defines, obtains, analyses and reports information in a way that enables and supports timely decision-making.

Require the use of indicators to assess the performance, procedures and results of security measures.

Review and evaluate the reports required for the whole area and for each department.

Use a process to resolve identified security issues and assign specific security tasks to appropriate individuals or sub-committees to take corrective action.

Issue quarterly reports on the results of security measures and security committee activities to the board of directors, managers, heads of departments and others responsible for monitoring security activities.

Establish strategies to enable the hospital to comply with national and international standards and requirements.

Evaluate the feasibility and effectiveness of corrective action plans and monitor them once completed.

Review and approve all security policies and procedures before they are adopted, and review them annually thereafter.

Summary of the research structure: brief explanation of the chapters.

This research is organised follows: In the introduction we find the research background, the problem statement using macro, meso and micro parameters, formulation and delimitation of the problem, the object of the research and field of action, as well as the general and specific objectives and the idea to be defended, concluding with the methodology to be used (methods, tools).

In Chapter I, the theoretical foundation is related to the topic of intervention plan to prevent occupational risks, for which the following concepts and terms are presented: Management of health services, Intervention plan, Occupational risks, among other topics.

In Chapter II, the methodological framework and the proposal's approach are described, the methodological procedure for the development of the research is described, and the proposal to solve the problem is presented.

In chapter IIIthe proposed alternative solution and its testing is presented and validated by experts with extensive knowledge of the research carried out.

CHAPTER I
THEORETICAL FRAMEWORK

1.1. Legal basis

The state has a broad legal and regulatory framework related to the guarantee of the right to health, the structuring of the National Health System and the protection of population groups. The mission of the Ministry of Labour is to coordinate the implementation of the Institutional Health and Safety and the Health and Safety Management System of the Ministry of Labour. It advises, trains, controls and monitors occupational risk prevention programmes in workplaces in order to reduce occupational accidents, improve productivity and the quality of life of workers.

1.1.1. Regulation of the Andean Safety and Health at Work Instrument

Resolution 957, in Chapter II, on Occupational Risk Prevention Policy, Article 4, in the framework of their National Occupational Safety and Health Systems, Member Countries shall promote the improvement of occupational safety and health conditions, in order to prevent damage to the physical and mental integrity of workers resulting from, related to or occurring during work. (Andean Community, 2005). In order to fulfil this obligation, each Member Country shall develop, implement and periodically review its national policy for the improvement of occupational safety and health conditions.

1.1.2. Constitution of the Republic of Ecuador

The constitution approved in 2008 constitutes the normative framework that governs the organisation and democratic life of the country, it represents a new social pact for the guarantee and exercise of rights and responsibilities in terms of the achievement of good living, the Sumak Kawsay. (constituent, 2008). In Chapter II, Section 7, Article 32 states that, "Health is a right guaranteed by the State, whose realisation is linked to the exercise of other rights, including the right to water, food, education, physical culture, work, social security, healthy environments and others that support good living. (Constituent Assembly, 2008).

Our country is committed to complying with its own laws, those that are typified in the Political Constitution of Ecuador (2008), in its Sixth Chapter: Work and Production, Third Section: Forms of Work and its Remuneration, ART. 326, where the right to work is based on the principles mentioned in numbers 5 and 6; and to all international law in force on Health and Safety, as a member of the Andean Community of Nations (CAN), it is obliged to comply with the provisions of the Andean Instrument on Safety and Health at Work, and its implementing regulations. It is an obligation for companies or institutions to have approved Internal Regulations for Health and Safety at Work (institutions with more than 10 workers) and its elaboration will be in accordance with the Ministerial Agreement 0220/05.

14

1.1.3. Organic Law of Health

The country also has several laws and has signed international agreements that have do with the guarantee of health rights such as: Organic Law on Health, where Article 6 states, "It is the responsibility of the Ministry of Public Health; To design and implement comprehensive and quality care programmes for people during all stages of life and in accordance with their particular conditions." (MAIS-FCI, 2018)

A priority axis of intervention is defined for the health sector: Strengthening disease prevention, control and surveillance: strengthening the epidemiological surveillance system, reinforcing prevention systems and comprehensive care for the main health problems and the capacity for immediate response to emergencies, contingencies and disasters. (MAIS-FCI, 2018).

1.2. Management of health services.

One of the main commitments of the state is to provide public services to the community and to guarantee equity, efficiency, effectiveness, quality and economy in their provision. However, given the deficient fulfilment of these guarantees, since the 1980s, both in developed countries and in those with dependent economies, a series of guidelines have been given for the provision of public services (Molina, 2009). (Molina, 2009).

Exchanges in health system management have occurred as part of public sector reforms, which have flourished in response to multiple national and international political, social, economic and technical-scientific forces. These changes seek to lead institutions towards the implementation of management models capable of responding efficiently and effectively to the changing needs of society in health services. (Molina, 2009).

1.2.1. What is Gestión?

According to Angélica Román in 2012, management means directing, administering resources, and achieving the proposed objectives and goals. This requires coordinating and motivating, properly articulating both the people and the material resources of an organisation or health institution so that these objectives are achieved in a context of effectiveness and efficiency. (Román, 2012). Management in the field of health can be divided into three main levels, which are as follows:

1.2.1.1. Macro management or regulatory management.

It refers to health policy and the role of the State, which is provided by the Ministry of Public Health of Ecuador as the highest health authority (AS), with the purpose steering, regulation, national planning and control. To meet the objectives of the MAIS-FCI, it organises and builds processes in order to define health services at the three levels of care, whose mission is the comprehensive care of individuals, families and communities in a given population space (MAIS-FCI, 2018). (MAIS-FCI, 2018).

In this area it is given in accordance with the principles of equity, universality, solidarity, quality and efficiency, determined in the promotion and prevention of population and occupational health.

1.2.1.2. Meso management or management of networks.

It is the articulation of facilities of differentiated complexity for the fulfilment of health objectives. It includes coordination between the various specialised and speciality hospitals and general hospitals, which must offer a defined portfolio of services incorporating preventive, promotional, curative and rehabilitative actions in order to achieve the health goals set for the country.At the managerial level, its management model is based on the planning, control and coordination of health services. Containing information and feedback on all current programmes in the health services, as well as occupational health at work.

1.2.1.3. Micro-management or clinical management .

It is provided at the first level of management in the health services, whether these are basic hospitals, in type A, B and C health units. Being the gateway as providers of health services in the country. (MAIS-FCI, 2018)

1.2.2.   Trends in the management of health services.

Since the 1970s and with greater emphasis in the 1980s, health systems have been on the agenda of governments and have been the subject of permanent analysis and reforms that have involved the development of new models for the provision of more and better services for a larger number of the population. These changes in the system are part of public sector reforms as a whole and have been initiated in developed countries and later in those with dependent economies, seeking greater efficiency, equity, economy, effectiveness and quality of health services. (Molina, 2009)

In these changes in the public health system, management is fundamentally oriented towards creating new paradigms centred on:

✓ Achieve greater equity in accessibility to health services.
✓ Achieve financial soundness of the system to ensure sustainability of services.
✓ Achieve greater efficiency, effectiveness and quality in the provision of services.
✓ Emphasise user-orientation, creating new cultural values in health organisations.
✓ Create incentives based on performance and results.
✓ Strengthen interdisciplinary and intersectoral teamwork.
✓ Generate an internal market and create competition (Molina, 2009).

1.2.4. Management models organisational.

The new trends arising from the new public administration and health system reforms imply new management styles, new ways of financing the system, so that it achieves the objectives and goals set and meets the needs of the community.
The management of services implies a broad knowledge of the components involved in the system. These components are:

1.2.4.1. Forms of funding

✓ Public financing based on taxes collected at central and local level, based on the Beveridge model, used in countries such as the UK, New Zealand, Italy, Spain and Cuba.
✓ Public funding based on compulsory social security contributions plus a percentage of taxes, based on the Bismarckian model used in countries such as Germany,
✓ The Netherlands, France, Belgium and in some Latin American countries, such as Argentina, Brazil, Ecuador, Colombia, Peru and Chile.
✓ Private funding based on voluntary insurance or direct payment services, used in the United States of America.

1.2.4.2. Payment methods for services.

✓ Capitation: stimulates disease prevention and health promotion, decreases demand for curative care and increases coverage.
✓ : high risk of over-utilisation of services.

✓ Fixed budgets: do not stimulate efficiency but control spending.
✓ Others: through vouchers, co-payments, moderator fees, etc.

1.2.4.3.   Service packages according to groups population.

It implies the definition of packages of services, which are shaped under cost-effectiveness criteria and, in some cases, differential packages according to the population group.

1.2.4.4. Policy Decentralisation

It has been identified as one of the central aspects of any current agenda in the field of health organisations. Different forms of decentralisation, deconcentration, delegation, devolution and privatisation are recognised. The aim is to make the state more efficient and effective, to strengthen democracy and the development of local governments and participation of social groups. It also gives autonomy to public hospitals managed by local, district or regional boards.

1.2.4.5. Internal reform of health organisations.

The reform of institutions and their development is essential for the achievement of goals, since it is through them that intervention strategies or plans materialise. They must implement better management styles with new administrative techniques to increase the efficiency, quality and effectiveness of services.

1.2.4.6. Improving the performance of employees in the public sector .

The aim is to employ fewer and better paid staff by creating performance-related incentives, improving job descriptions, etc.

1.2.4.7. Citizen participation .

The participation of different groups, organisations, associations, etc. is promoted as a mechanism to strengthen democratic processes, create forms of community participation in decision-making and encourage citizen oversight. Likewise, to identify interest groups that may support or oppose public management (MAIS-FCI, 2018).

1.2.5.   Organisational models for the management of health services .

Based on the trends that have emerged with the new public administration, some authors such as Ferlie have identified four management models that are being implemented in public organisations. These models have influenced health organisations and, depending on the political, social and economic context, as well as the legislation in force, the level of health development, the objectives of the system and the needs of the community in each country, among others, each organisation tends more towards one of the models, although including some components of the others. (Ferlie, 2017).

- **The quest for efficiency**

✓ Increasing the volume of activities with the same resources. "Doing more with less
✓ Financial control
✓ Management control
✓ Audit
✓ Emphasis on customer service
✓ Less regulation

✓ Performance related payments
✓ Less influence and power of professional groups and trade unions
✓ Emphasis on leadership and managerial profiles (Ferlie, 2017).

- **Decentralisation and flexibility**
✓ Emphasis on marketing
✓ Shift from hierarchical administration to contracting and local development
✓ Elimination of administrative layers and reduction of human resources at central and intermediate levels of the organisations.
✓ Separation of insurers and service producers
✓ Change of management and control to new management styles
✓ Encouraging the formation of networks of organisations and strategic alliances
✓ Flexibility of management (Ferlie, 2017).

- **Pursuit of excellence**

✓ Strong focus on culture and organisational development: values, culture, rituals and symbols
✓ Emphasis on learning processes
✓ Change management based on employee and organisational values
✓ Humanistic approach stimulating self-development and participation
✓ Emphasis on charismatic and transformational leadership rather than transactional leadership (Ferlie, 2017).

- **Public service orientation**

✓ Merging public and private sector administrative styles
✓ Emphasis on the mission of the public sector as distinct from the private sector
✓ Raising administrative quality by involving private sector practices

✓ Ensuring social accountability of services

✓ Increased concern for quality of service

✓ Emphasis on the user and the relationship with citizenship

✓ Devolution of power to the local authority

✓ Scepticism in the public sector market (Ferlie, 2017).

1.3. Intervention Plan.

According to María José Fuster Ruiz de Apodaca Social Psychologist UNED, she defines an intervention plan as "Any social action, individual or group, aimed at producing changes in a given reality that involves and affects a given social group". According to Rodríguez Espinar, given his research in the 1990s, he defines an Intervention Plan as a set of systematic, planned actions, based on identified needs and oriented towards goals, as a response to those needs, with a supporting theory.

Features
✓ They are oriented towards the achievement of a specific objective.
✓ They combine human and non-human resources for the coordinated implementation of interrelated activities.
✓ Limited duration: they have a beginning and an end.

Life cycle of a project.

Creation of the project
a. Conceptual phase
b. Definition phase

Project implementation
a. Implementation phase
b. Completion phase

1.3.1. Phases or stages of an intervention plan .

Four phases are considered in the design of a project or intervention plan: 1:
Diagnosis and analysis of intervention needs.
2.- Second phase:
Planning and design of the components of the action plan.
3.- Third phase:
Implementation of the actions of the proposed plan.
4.- Fourth phase:
Formative (process) and summative (product) evaluation.

1.3.2. Conditions determining the intervention plans.

✓ The initiative is driven and sustained by a person or persons who are members of small groups that register, on a daily basis in the health institution, situations of conflict or tension; these situations are rarely communicated to management and, when they are, satisfactory responses are not obtained from them (Ambriz Tapia, 2018). (Ambriz Tapia, 2018).

✓ Institutional actions avoid the necessary spaces for analysis, criticism and reflection on the tasks carried out. It is common observe issues such as: scarcity of resources, lack of coordination, disputes over power, distancing from authority, etc.

✓ The analysis of the intervention begins with an understanding of the history of the institution in which the situation develops, the aspects that converge in the work, its origin, development, present day, the policies on which it is based, the relationships between the sub-systems present, the history of its members as a group and as individuals, the meaning they

give to their work and their relationship with the various institutional bodies.
✓ Preparing the actions themselves implies that, in accordance with the depth of understanding of the actions of the institutional context and, above all, with the knowledge of the group of observables to be intervened, the intervention plan does not violate the process with aversive breaks, but gradually transforms it, qualitatively from its own logic.
✓ Carry out the project's own actions within the necessary management and according to the natural resistance, which conditions the continuity of alternative practices.
✓ To open up spaces for analysis and criticism collective production, where participants maintain a proactive attitude, constructing the institution's own alternative action.

1.3.3. Diagnosis and needs analysis of intervention plans.

Any plan is supposed to be the result of reflection and analysis of needs, problematic situations or situations to be improved, from which solutions or proposals for action are determined. (Ambriz Tapia, 2018).

The needs assessment involves two phases:
✓ Identification: through reflection, "real" needs are identified.

✓ Prioritisation: priorities are set and resource allocation decisions are made.

1.3.4. Components of an intervention plan .

✓ Intervention Objectives (What for?).
✓ Content of the intervention (What?).
✓ Initial Situation and Development Context (Where?).
✓ Targets of the intervention and levels of action (individual, group, institutional, etc.) (Who?)
✓ Intervention Methodology (How?). (Ambriz Tapia, 2018)

1.3.5. Implementation of a plan for intervention.

✓ Application of the methodology.
✓ Project development and monitoring

1.3.6. Indicators for evaluating a plan for intervention.

✓ **Independence:** The same indicator should not be used to measure different objectives, each should have its own indicator.

✓ **Verifiability:** It must be possible to verify empirically the changes that occur with the project.
✓ **Validity:** Indicators must actually measure what they claim to measure.

✓ **Accessibility:** The data obtained through the indicators should be easy to obtain (Ambriz Tapia, 2018).

1.3.7. Integrated approach: the logical framework

Analytical tool for planning and management of projects oriented by objectives. Method with different steps from identification to formulation and its final result should be the project planning matrix (Fuster Ruiz, 2008).

Steps:

1.3.7.1. Identification stage a.- Analysis of participation:
✓ Analyse the social reality in which the project will intervene and examine its characteristics and particularities.

b.- Analysis of the problems:
Prioritise the problem:

✓ Identify existing problems

✓ Determining the most important (focal, central, main) problem: Precise and unambiguous Identify causes and effects of the prioritised problem:

✓ What is the problem (central problem)?
✓ What caused the problem (causes)
✓ What are consequences (effects)?
c.- Analysis of the objectives
✓ Describe the hypothetical situation if the problems were solved.

✓ Negative states in the problem diagram are transcribed into positive desirable states.
✓ Review of approaches to remove unrealistic or unnecessary objectives and add new ones if necessary.
✓ Key question: How can we solve the problem (ends and means)? d. - Analysis of alternatives

✓ Available resources
✓ Estimated time to achieve objectives
✓ Adequacy of the parties involved

✓ Risks and possibilities to achieve objectives

✓ Contribution of alternatives to broader objectives
✓ Effects/impacts
✓ Feasibility

1.3.7.2. Structure of design

Project planning
✓ Logical framework: A tool to strengthen design, implementation and evaluation of intervention plans or projects (Fuster Ruiz, 2008).

1.4. Risk

1.4.1. Basic conceptualisations

According to José Cortez in 2007, in his research on Techniques for the prevention of occupational risks, safety and hygiene in the workplace, occupational risk is defined as the existing dangers in our work tasks or in our own environment or workplace, which can cause accidents or any type of accidents which, in turn, are factors that can cause injuries, physical or psychological damage, trauma, etc. (Cortes, 2007). Whatever its possible effect, it is always negative for our health.

1.4.1.1. Risk.-

Likelihood of occurrence of harm as a result of exposure.

1.4.1.2. Conditions of work.

Any work characteristic that may have a significant influence on the generation of risks to the safety and health of workers (Cortes, 2007).
Damage arising from work
Illnesses, pathologies or injuries arising of or in connection with work. They may be:
Accidents at work. Occupational diseases.
Other work-related illnesses and pathologies (Cortes, 2007)

1.4.1.3. Health.

According to the World Health Organisation (WHO), in its 1948 constitution, health is defined as a state of complete physical, mental, spiritual, emotional and social well-being and not merely the absence of disease or infirmity.

1.4.1.4. Danger.

Thus, we can define hazard as the set of elements that, being present in working conditions, can trigger a decrease in ' health (Patón Jesús, 2021).

1.4.2. Factors risk.-

These are factors that are present in the work environment and are associated with the likelihood of an unfavourable health event (harm) occurring to us.
They are characteristic of the different production processes, and are sometimes associated with accidents or occupational illnesses or a host of other, less specific ailments (Patón Jesús, 2021).
Risk factors are directly related to or dependent on safety conditions. They will always have their origin in one of the following four aspects of work:
✓ Working premises (electrical installations, gas installations, fire prevention, ventilation, temperatures, etc.).
✓ Work organisation (physical and/or mental workload, organisation and organisation of work, monotony, repetitiveness, lack of creativity, isolation, participation, etc.).
✓ Type of activity (work equipment: computers, machines, tools, etc., storage and handling of loads, etc.).
✓ Raw materials (flammable materials, hazardous chemicals, etc.)

1.4.3. Biological risks

Biological risk is conditioned by exposure to biological agents: bacteria, fungi, viruses (hepatitis B, C, yellow fever, measles, mumps, HIV, dengue fever...), parasites (leishmania, tapeworm, toxoplasma...), spores, recombination products, human or animal cell cultures and potentially infectious biological agents that these cells may contain, such as prions, as well as various types of toxins. (Patón Jesús, 2021).

1.4.3.1. Classification of biological agents

Group 1:
Agents unlikely to cause disease in humans. Group 2:
Agents that can cause disease in humans and may pose a hazard to those who work, are unlikely to spread to the community and effective prophylaxis or treatment is generally available.
Group 3:
Agents that can cause serious disease in humans and present a serious hazard to those who work, with a risk of spreading to the community and generally effective prophylaxis or

treatment available.

Group 4:

Agents that cause serious disease in humans and pose a serious danger to those who work, with a high likelihood of spreading to the community and generally without effective prophylaxis or treatment (Patón Jesús, 2021).

1.4.3.2. entry

These agents can enter our body through different routes:

Respiratory:

Organisms in the environment enter our bodies when we breathe, we talk, we cough...

Digestive:

They can come into contact by eating, drinking or accidental ingestion by passing into the mouth, oesophagus, stomach and intestines.

Dermal:

By contact with the skin, increasing the likelihood of access when the skin is wounded or poorly preserved.

Parenteral:

Through blood or mucous membranes: contact with eyes or mouth, punctures, cuts.

1.4.3.3. Preventive measures: Universal Precautions

So-called "universal precautions" are the fundamental strategy for occupational risk prevention against all blood-borne micro-organisms.Staff members will have to apply the fundamental principle that all samples should be handled as if they were infectious. Compliance with one universal precaution does not exempt or exclude you from following or performing the others (Patón Jesús, 2021).

These are universal precautions:

• Vaccination (active immunisation)

• Personal hygiene rules:

a) Cover hand wounds and injuries with waterproof dressing when starting work. Avoid direct exposure when there are injuries that cannot be covered.

b) Do not wear rings, bracelets, chains or other jewellery.

c) Hand washing should be carried out at the beginning and end of the day, and after any technique that may involve contact with infectious material. This washing should be carried out with water and liquid soap, except in special situations in which antimicrobial substances should be used (Patón Jesús, 2021).

After hand washing, hands shall be dried with disposable paper towels or air flow.
d) Do not eat, drink, wear make-up or smoke in the work area.
e) Do not pipette by mouth.
• Barrier protection elements:
f) Gloves.
g) Masks.
h) Gowns.
i) Eye protection.
• Care with sharp or pointed objects:

j) Take precautions when using sharps, needles and syringes, and after use, as well as in cleaning and disposal procedures.
k) Do not encapsulate needles or sharps or subject them to any manipulation.
l) Sharps (needles, syringes and other sharp instruments) shall be placed in appropriate containers with safety lids to prevent their loss during transport, close to the workplace and avoid overfilling.
m) Healthcare personnel handling sharp objects shall be responsible for their disposal.
• Proper sterilisation and disinfection of instruments and surfaces.
• Proper waste disposal.
• Reporting accidents as soon as possible and following the relevant protocol.

1.4.4. Risks chemicals

Chemical substances are present in the daily activity of the health sector. The storage, handling and management of their waste entail multiple risks that can seriously affect the health of workers (Patón, 2021).

Chemicals

Chemical agent: Defines chemical agent as any chemical element or compound, alone or in a mixture, as it occurs in its natural state or is produced, used or discharged, including discharge as waste, in an occupational activity, whether intentionally produced or not and whether intentionally placed on the market or not. (Patón, 2021).

Hazardous chemical agent: A chemical agent that may represent a risk to the safety and health of workers due to its physicochemical, chemical or toxicological properties and the way it is used or present in the workplace.

Health effects

Exposure to hazardous substances or chemicals is characterised by being of low intensity (low concentrations) but of long duration, and can even cover all or a large part of a worker's working life. This means that the effects appear in the long term, after years or decades of exposure, and that their evolution is very slow (insidious), taking a long time for the symptoms of the affectation to manifest themselves.

These are chronic degenerative diseases, with long periods of evolution (latency) and which manifest themselves at a later age, such as solvent toxic encephalopathy or the various cancers caused by chemical agents and hazardous substances.

1.4.5. Risks physical

Among the physical risks, which also include noise and vibrations, in the health sector we highlight exposure to electromagnetic energy or radiation (Patón Jesús, 2021). In healthcare workplaces, we may be exposed a wide range of these physical agents: Ionising radiation used in radiodiagnosis, interventional radiology and radiotherapy (linear accelerators); magnetic fields associated with nuclear magnetic resonance or rehabilitation equipment; infrared, short wave and microwaves also used in rehabilitation; lasers used in surgery, ophthalmology, dermatology or rehabilitation; UV light used in the sterilisation of clinical equipment, phototherapy and photocopiers; the proliferation of mobile telephones; the use of radioactive radiation in the treatment of cancer; the use of radioactive radiation in the treatment of patients with cancer; the use of radioactive radiation in the treatment of patients with cancer; the use of radioactive radiation in the treatment of patients with cancer; the use of radioactive radiation in the treatment of patients with cancer and in the treatment of patients with cancer.between workers, patients and users; cordless phones; wi-fi; welding equipment that can emit ultraviolet, visible or infrared radiation, etc.

1.4.6. Risks ergonomic

Ergonomic risks are mainly associated with musculoskeletal injuries, which are the most frequent occupational diseases and the first cause of permanent disability (Patón Jesús, 2021). Musculoskeletal disorders include a large number of injuries to muscles, tendons, nerves, joints, ligaments, etc., usually located in the back, neck, shoulders, elbows and wrists.

They can be caused by a single sufficient strain (accidents) or by the sum of several strains with cumulative effects (work-related diseases and the cause of a small group of occupational diseases). The predominant symptom is pain, muscle contracture, inflammation and decreased or impaired function of the affected area. The causes of injuries derived from ergonomic risks can be varied: adopting inadequate and forced postures, repetitive movements, handling loads and patients or working with data display screens in inadequate ergonomic conditions (Patón Jesús, 2021).

Ergonomic hazards are mainly caused by:

•Manual handling of loads:
The mobilisation of the sick is one of the most frequent tasks in the health sector.

• Postural hygiene:
Correct postural hygiene is essential to avoid injuries when carrying out any activity and even more so in the case of handling loads.

• Forced movements:
With or without load, they can lead to muscle contractures and joint and ligament injuries.

• Sedentary lifestyle:
Lack of physical activity and sedentary lifestyles lead to muscle weakness and are an added risk factor.

• Unforeseen movements:
If the patient makes an unexpected sudden movement, it is necessary for the worker to overexert him/herself, and this is usually done quickly and with inappropriate posture, which increases the risk of injury.

1.4.7. Risks psychosocial

Psychosocial risks are the specific risks to which workers are exposed due to poor organisation at work and which generate negative health . (Patón Jesús, 2021)

Risk factors

Psychosocial risk factors are all those aspects related to the design, organisation and management of work that can cause damage to the health of workers.
These factors include:

• More work than we can do in the allotted time (lack of staff or technical or material means).

• Our work requires a great deal of intellectual effort (making decisions, controlling many things at once, etc.) or of the senses (requiring a great deal of concentration, precision and skill), without the necessary resources.

• Contact users and patients with transferential processes of emotions or feelings are established.

• Having to hide emotions, feelings and opinions.

• Not receiving adequate help from superiors and colleagues to get the job done.

• Working in conditions of isolation or conditions that prevent or hinder sociability.

• Absence of teams and group feeling (Patón Jesús, 2021).

Health effects

The effects of exposure to psychosocial risks are manifested :
Stress: Inadequate fit between the individual and the work environment due to both the demands of the work reality that must be met by the individual and the demands of the individual that must be met by the work reality.
Burnout: This is a response to chronic work-related stress made up of negative attitudes and feelings towards the people with whom one works and towards one's own professional role, as well as the experience of being emotionally exhausted. It occurs mainly in professions that work with people (Patón Jesús, 2021).

1.5. Partial conclusions of chapter.

In the country, the mission of the Ministry of Labour is to coordinate the execution of the Institutional in Safety and Health and the Safety and Health Management System of the Ministry of Labour Relations. To advise, train, control and follow up on occupational risk prevention programmes in workplaces with the aim of reducing occupational accidents, improving productivity and the quality of life of workers.
Our country is committed to complying with the laws that typified in the Political Constitution of Ecuador (2008), in its Sixth Chapter: Work and Production, Third Section: Forms of Work and its Remuneration.
To manage is to direct, to administer resources, to achieve the proposed objectives and goals. Management, in the field of health, can be divided into three main levels, which are as follows:
Macro management or regulatory management: This refers to health policy and the role of the State, which is provided by the Ministry of Public Health of Ecuador as the highest health authority.
Meso management or network management: This includes the articulation of facilities of differentiated complexity for the fulfilment of health objectives.
Micro-management or clinical management: This is given to care at the first level of management in health services.
According to María José Fuster Ruiz de Apodaca Social Psychologist UNED, she defines an intervention plan as "Any social action, individual or group, aimed at producing changes in a given reality that involves and affects a given social group".
The phases of an intervention plan are: diagnosis, planning, implementation and evaluation.

Occupational risk is defined as hazards in our work or in our own environment or workplace, which can cause accidents or any type of accidents which, in turn, are factors that can cause injuries, physical or psychological damage, trauma, etc.
It is clear that a risk is the likelihood of harm as a result exposure.
Risk factors include: biological risks, chemical risks, physical risks, ergonomic risks, psychosocial risks.

CHAPTER II.

METHODOLOGICAL FRAMEWORK

2.1. DESCRIPTION OF THE METHODOLOGICAL PROCEDURE FOR THE DEVELOPMENT OF THE INVESTIGATION

The characteristics of the research will be qualitative-quantitative, with the quantitative aspect being fundamental. The qualitative characteristics of the existing problem are determined on the basis of observation and permanent dialogue with those involved in the problematic situation. The quantitative aspects are ratified by statistically tabulating the results of the field research carried out on the respective population.

The design this research is considered longitudinal as it assessed the evolution of phenomena and trends, examined changes over time, collected data, described variables and analysed incidence and interrelationships at different points in time.

The current research was based on bibliographical studies and field work, using books and the internet as a source, as well as up-to-date information from authors who are experts in their field, which helped to achieve the results of the research.

2.1.1. TYPES OF RESEARCH

2.1.1.1. Bibliography.

Established in the research of existing information in books, magazines and the Internet, it will be very useful to elaborate the theoretical framework that scientifically supports the solution to the problem. This enquiry makes it possible, among other things, to support the research to be carried out, to avoid undertaking research that has already been carried out, to learn from experiments that have already been carried out in order to repeat them when necessary, to continue interrupted or incomplete research or in search of suggestive information.

2.1.1.2. From the field.

Produced at the limit in the area where the indications of the problem are generated, for this specific case it will be carried out in the Canton of Santa Elena, Province of Santa Elena.

2.1.1.3. Descriptive.

The purpose of descriptive research is to gain insight into prevailing situations, customs and attitudes through the accurate description of activities, objects, processes and people. Its purpose is not limited to data collection but to the prediction and identification relationships between two or more variables.

2.1.2. Population and sample.

2.1.2.1. Universe

The population or universe to be considered corresponds to the Nursing Staff of the General Hospital Dr. Liborio Panchana Sotomayor of the Santa Elena Canton (9 nurses).

2.1.2.2. Research sample.

In order to determine the sample size of the research universe, sampling is used, and the formula is applied where the total population is established for the collection of information. However, in the present research, the population is made up of 9 nurses from whom the information will be collected using the research instruments.

2.1.3. Methods, techniques and instruments of research.

2.1.3.1. Methods

The research methods allowed us to carry out the research in the right way and thus we were able to find the results we had set out.
The research methods to be used are:

2.1.3.1.1.   Inductive - Deductive.

Inductive research explores particular aspects in order to arrive at a general understanding of the subject under investigation; it starts from a general knowledge of the subject and goes on to investigate its particularities.

2.1.3.1.2.   Analytical - synthetic.

"This method involves analysis, i.e. the separation of a whole into its parts or into theirconstituent elements. It is based on the fact that in order to understand a phenomenon it is necessary to break it down into its parts. It involves synthesis (from the Greek synthesis, which means the union of elements to form a whole).

2.1.3.2. research techniques.

Data collection is the special activity of collecting, processing or analysing data that is carried out with a certain orientation and with the support of interviews and surveys.

2.1.3.2.1. Interview.

It was used to collect information verbally, through questions posed by the analyst. Respondents may be managers or employees who are current users of the existing system, potential users of the proposed system, or those who will provide data or be affected by proposed application the interview guide.

2.1.3.2.2. Survey

A quantitative technique consisting of research conducted on a sample of subjects, representative of a larger group, carried out in the context of everyday life, using standardised questioning procedures in order to obtain quantitative measurements on a large number of objective and subjective characteristics of the population.

2.1.3.2.3. The observation.

This technique will be developed by appreciating the particularities of the problem, with the help of this instrument the researcher will be able to understand the case study in order to have a more accurate appreciation of what is happening.

2.2. CHARACTERISATION OF THE SECTOR, BRANCH, COMPANY, INSTITUTIONAL CONTEXT OR PROBLEM SELECTED FOR THE RESEARCH.

General Hospital Dr. Liborio Panchana Sotomayor, with a modern structure and state-of-the-art technology, second level of care with a capacity of 120 beds, located:
In the Province of Santa Elena, Canton Santa Elena, Márquez de La Plata Avenue, in front of the general cemetery.
Within its capacity for resolution, we can mention the institutional portfolio of services: Outpatient Clinic, with the different services and programmes existing in the Ministry of Public Health, Emergency (triage), Hospitalisation (internal medicine, surgery, paediatrics, maternity, newborns), ICU, Surgical and Obstetric Centre, clinical laboratory and imaging, administrative areas and the area of the present investigation, sterilisation, which has the latest instruments and equipment, in which 9 nurses work on a rotating schedule.

2.3. ANALYSIS AND INTERPRETATION OF THE RESULTS OF THE APPLICATION OF THE SURVEY CARRIED OUT ON THE NURSING STAFF IN THE STERILISATION AREA.

Once the surveys had been applied, the following information was obtained:

1. Knowledge of a Manual of Procedures-Protocols for the prevention of occupational risks in sterilisation?

CATEGORY	# USERS	%
Yes	3	33
No	6	67
Total	9	100%

Prepared by: Authors
Source: Survey

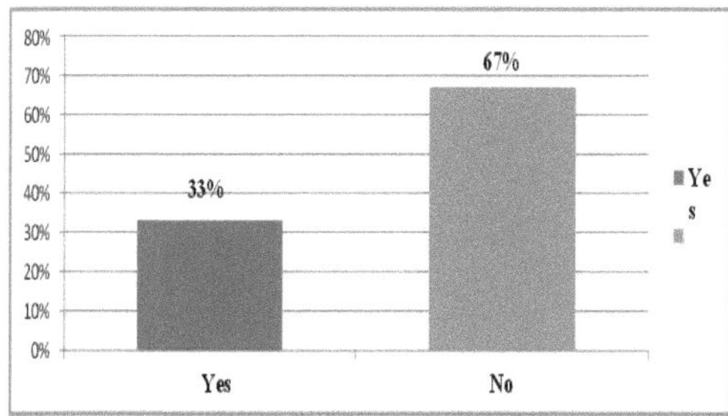

Prepared by: Authors
Source: Survey.

Analysis:

In the sterilisation area there is no occupational risk manual, which means that the personnel working in this area are totally unaware of the risks they may suffer during their working hours, as there is a lack of concern on the part of the area leader to provide or produce an occupational risk manual for the personnel on causes of the risks, as evidenced in the survey of the nursing personnel (67%).

2. Does the hospital unit have a sterilisation quality and occupational risk prevention committee?

CATEGORY	# USERS	%
Yes	2	22
No	7	78
Total	9	100%

Prepared by: Authors
Source: Survey

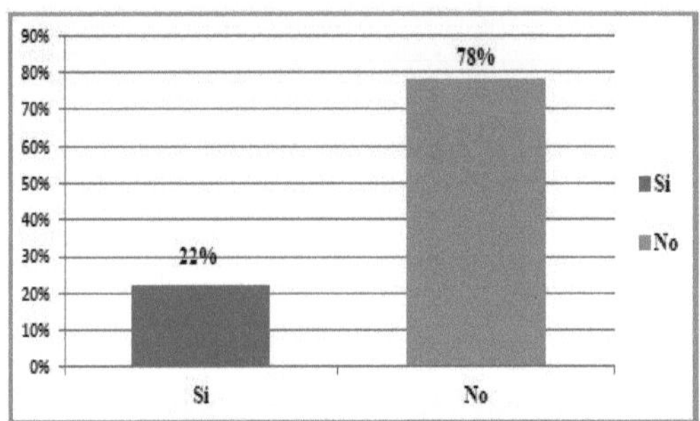

Prepared by: Authors
Source: Survey.

Analysis:

It can be shown that 78% of the staff stated that there no occupational risk committee in the hospital unit, and that the management-administrative staff have not yet received any training or knowledge about occupational risk manuals so that the staff working in the health unit have the preventive measures to avoid future occupational risks.

3. Identification of occupational risk factors in the sterilisation area?

CATEGORY	# Yes	%	# No	%	TOTAL	
Chemicals	6	67%	3	33%	9	100%
Ergonomic	8	89%	1	11%	9	100%
Physicists	7	78%	2	22%	9	100%
Biologicals	7	78%	2	22%	9	100%
Psychosocial	9	100%	0	0%	9	100%

Prepared by: Authors
Source: Survey

34

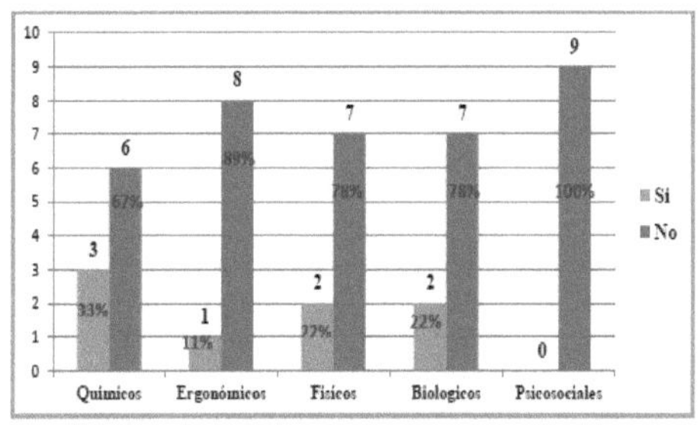

Prepared by: Authors
Source: Survey.

Analysis:

Under the survey it can be shown that 82% of the staff in the sterilisation area do not have the respective knowledge about the accidents and risk factors that can occur in this area due to the lack of training and the carelessness of the staff in charge without awareness of the risks.

4. Are systems or circulation routes in the sterilisation area well lit?

CATEGORY	# USERS	%
Yes	8	89
No	1	11
Total	9	100%

Prepared by: Authors
Source: Survey

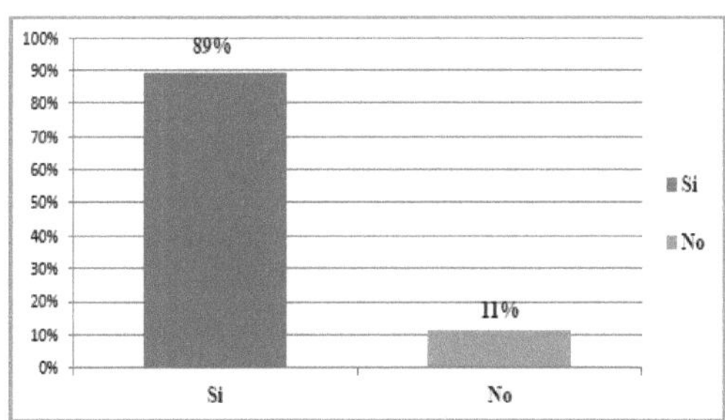

Prepared by: Authors
Source: Survey.

35

Analysis:

In the sterilisation area, 89% of the nursing staff say that they have perfect lighting, as the maintenance staff carry out their respective checks to prevent defects in the lighting.

5. Are materials and means of protection available to protect against accidents in the sterilisation area?

ATEGORY	# USERS	%
Yes	4	44
No	5	56
Total	9	100%

Prepared by: Authors
Source: Survey

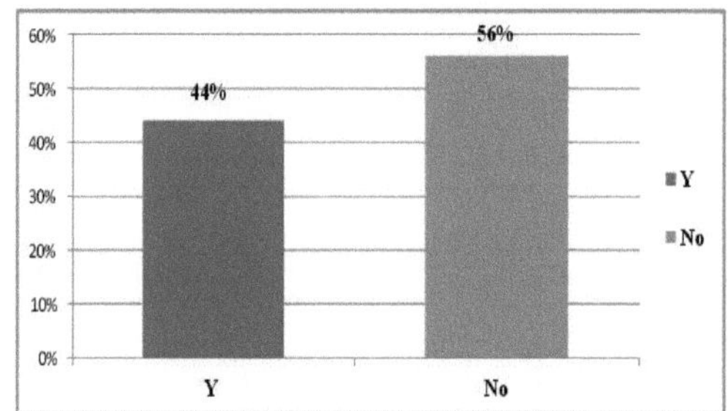

Prepared by: Authors
Source: Survey.

Analysis:

The area does not have protection material in the event of an accident at work and due to lack of knowledge, they do not use protective equipment for their work activities in the sterilisation area, as these are useful implements for preventing accidents in the future, as evidenced by the survey carried out, where it was found that 56% do not have protective equipment.

6. Regular removal of stains or residues of hazardous substances or contaminants in the sterilisation area?

CATEGORY	# USERS	%
Yes	3	33
No	6	67
Total	9	100%

Prepared by: Authors
Source: Survey

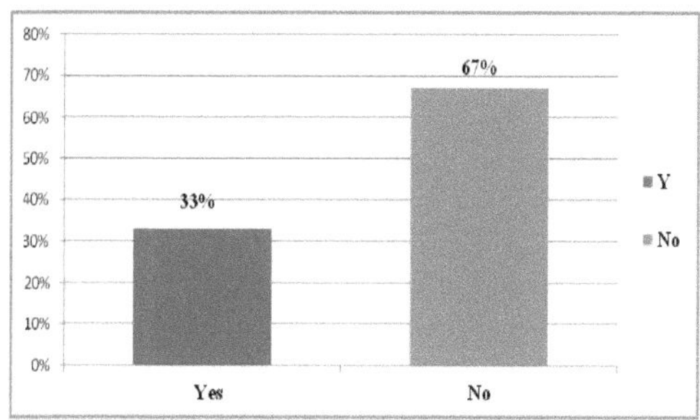

Prepared by: Authors
Source: Survey.

Analysis:

The elimination of contaminating waste is not carried out on a regular basis, as the personnel lack training in order to have the necessary knowledge and thus avoid contamination in the sterilisation area, aggravating the problem of the eminent occupational risks for the integrity of each person in the aforementioned area. 67% of the personnel do not carry out regular elimination.

7. Accidents with short sharp material cuts and/or punctures?

CATEGORY	# USERS	%
Yes	4	44
No	5	56
Total	9	100%

Prepared by: Authors
Source: Survey

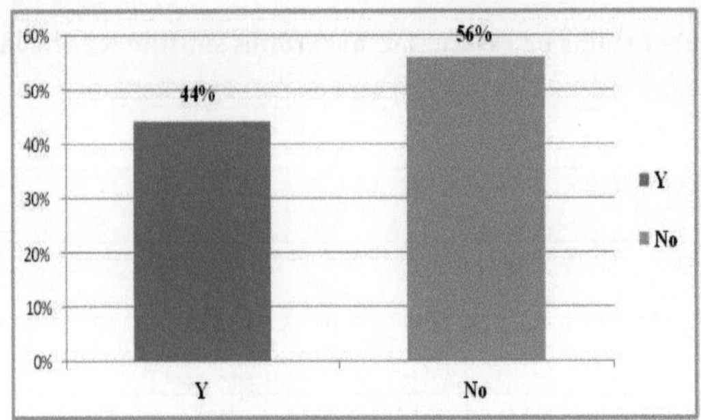

Prepared by: Authors
Source: Survey.

Analysis:

The associated indicators in the sterilisation area are not easily visualised, so that the personnel have the power to carry out their work safely when counting the equipment and wrapping it in order to avoid future errors. Occupational accidents occur on average among nursing staff, with 44% of staff indicating that they have suffered occupational accidents involving cuts and/or punctures. Due to the lack of knowledge about norms and standards in the handling of sterilisation equipment and instruments, there is a risk of accidents at work.

8. Training on the handling of sterilisation equipment and its ?

CATEGORY	# USERS	%
Yes	5	56
No	4	44
Total	9	100%

Prepared by: Authors
Source: Survey

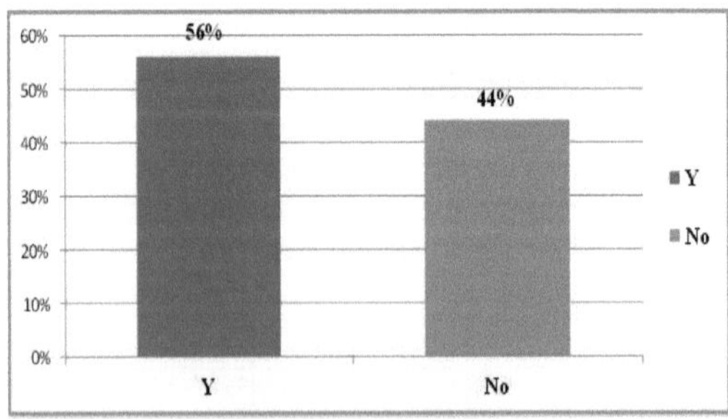

Prepared by: Authors
Source: Survey.

Analysis:

In the sterilisation area, the personnel have received training on the handling of autoclaves and sterilisers from the suppliers, as these instruments are very important in order to avoid occupational hazards in this area, thus raising the awareness of the personnel in order to avoid occupational hazards in the aforementioned area.

9. Knowledge of the nursing staff's instructions for action in an accident with biological, chemical or other material?

CATEGORY	# USERS	%
Yes	3	33
No	6	67
Total	9	100%

Prepared by: Authors
Source: Survey

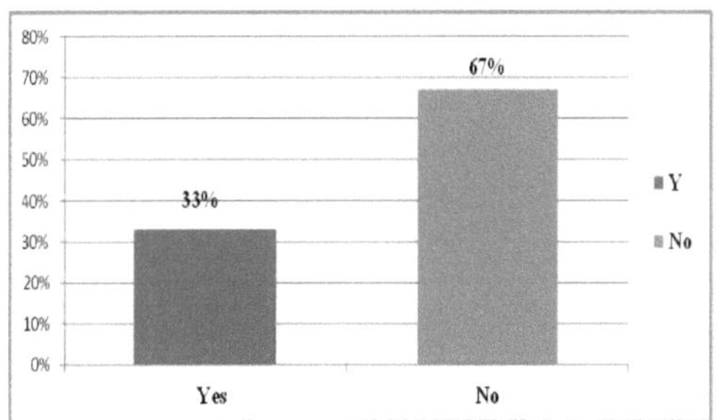

Prepared by: Authors
Source: Survey.

Analysis:

It is important to know the lack of knowledge of the nursing staff about the procedure for action in the event of an accident with biological, chemical or other materials. 67% of the nurses indicate that they do not know about the procedure they should follow in the event of suffering this type of accident.

10. Existence of conflicts between nursing staff in the sterilisation area?

CATEGORY	# USERS	%
Yes	3	33
No	6	67
Total	9	100%

Prepared by: Authors
Source: Survey

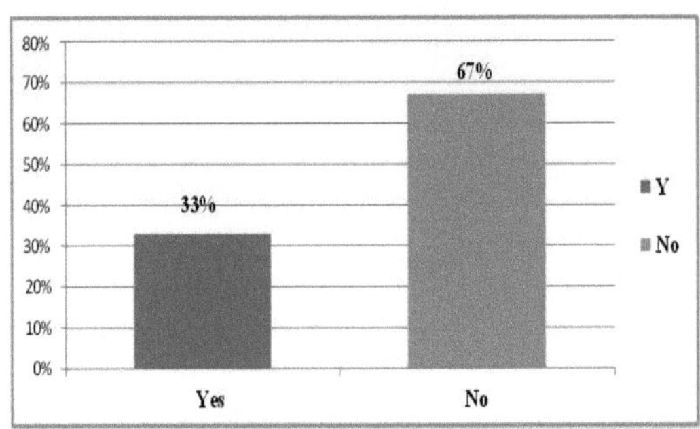

Prepared by: Authors
Source: Survey.

Analysis:

There is no conflict among the nursing staff in the sterilisation area, 67% of whom are not trained to avoid occupational hazards, but they work as a team to improve this area, although they are unaware of some of the factors that can lead to accidents at work.

11. Does the hospital unit have an intervention plan to prevent occupational hazards in the sterilisation area?

CATEGORY	# USERS	%
Yes	1	11
No	8	89
Total	9	100%

Prepared by: Authors
Source: Survey

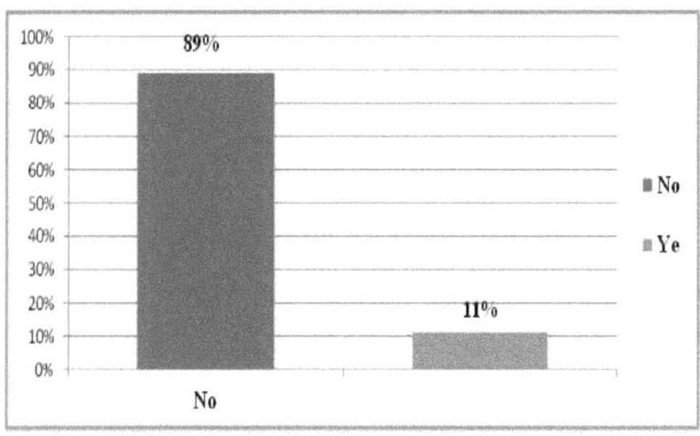

Prepared by: Authors
Source: Survey.

Analysis:

With all that has been explained and analysed above, it is evident that there is no intervention plan in the health unit to prevent occupational hazards, due to the lack of management in the improvement of the area and the implementation of strategies to identify the factors, which should be socialised. In addition, insist on training in the handling of equipment and instruments, in order to take the corresponding decisions with knowledge.

Occupational risk in the health institution.

The General Hospital Dr. Liborio Panchana Sotomayor, in the sterilisation area consists of 9 nurses with a rotating timetable, where there is a problem of lack of knowledge to avoid occupational hazards, where the staff have been working in this area for years, and where the following has been identified:

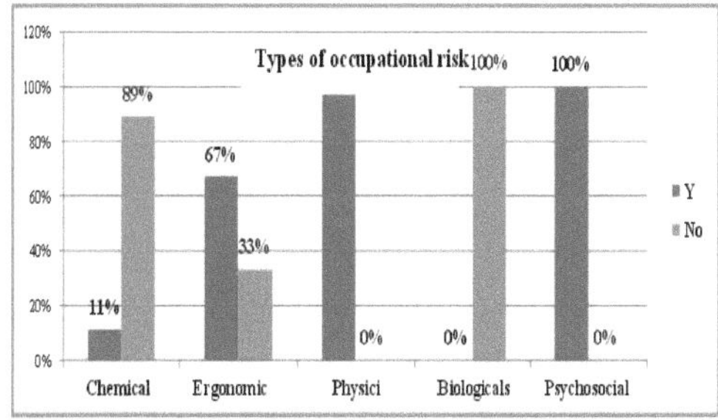

Prepared by: Authors
Source: Survey.

Analysis:

Of the nine (9) nurses who work in the sterilisation area, at least one has suffered an accident with a **chemical** (antiseptic), due to the lack of knowledge and awareness of the use of protective equipment.

Among the **ergonomic** risks, six (6) nurses have reported pain and discomfort due to frequent and rapid movement when transporting the material to be sterilised or sterilised, **physical risks** (all have suffered at least one superficial burn when handling instruments), and in terms of **psychosocial** risks, nine (9) nurses report a lack of organisation and an intervention plan in terms of frequent training to improve the level of knowledge in the management of the sterilisation area. In terms of biological risks, none of the nurses have so far reported this.

Interpretation of the results

From the universe surveyed (nursing staff), information was obtained that indicates that the problem, its causes and effects exist, as well as the possible solution of an intervention plan to avoid occupational risk in the sterilisation area in the General Hospital Dr. Liborio Panchana Sotomayor, Canton Santa Elena, Santa Elena Province, in order to avoid occupational risk and accidents in the sterilisation area. In this way it is expressed that the research is evident and the idea to be defended is confirmed.

2.4. VALIDATION OR VERIFICATION OF THE IDEA TO DEFEND.

This is validated by the results of the following questions: question one of the survey conducted shows that there is no manual of procedures for occupational risk prevention protocols in the sterilisation area, question two of the survey conducted shows the lack of a quality and occupational risk prevention committee and the need for a training plan in the aforementioned area, Question three of the survey shows that they do not know or are not clear about the most frequent occupational risk factors that cause problems and make it necessary to have a training plan on occupational risks. Liborio Panchana Sotomayor Hospital.

2.5. RESEARCHER'S PROPOSAL: MODEL, SYSTEM, METHODOLOGY, PROCEDURE, AMONG OTHERS, CARRIED OUT BY THE RESEARCHER.

Based on the theory of authors in biosafety standards and occupational risk, an intervention plan is proposed: Intervention Plan to avoid occupational risk in the sterilisation area of the General Hospital Dr. Liborio Panchana Sotomayor, Santa Elena canton, Santa Elena Province.

2.6. Partial conclusions of chapter.

✓ The field research supported the problem through the application of surveys directed at nurses in the sterilisation area of the General Hospital Dr. Liborio Panchana Sotomayor, the information obtained from which will be useful for the development of the proposal.

✓ Most of the nurses agree that there are no processes in place in the hospital for the management of skills and abilities to avoid occupational risk in the sterilisation area.

✓ It was possible to identify that there are factors such as the non-periodic elimination of waste or means of protection to avoid occupational risk, as this has been done empirically and on a daily basis due to the lack of training, awareness and a manual of procedures and protocols for the prevention of occupational risks in sterilisation.

✓ With the results of the survey, the idea to defend was verified, since an intervention plan is needed to prevent work-related accidents among the nursing staff working at the General Hospital, through the implementation of occupational risk training.

CHAPTER III
PROPOSAL AND VALIDATION

3.1. Proposal.

INTERVENTION PLAN TO PREVENT OCCUPATIONAL HAZARDS IN THE STERILISATION AREA OF THE GENERAL HOSPITAL DR. LIBORIO PANCHANA SOTOMAYOR GENERAL HOSPITAL, SANTA ELENA CANTON, SANTA ELENA PROVINCE.

3.1.1. Location of the proposed .

The present proposal is located in the Province of Santa Elena, Santa Elena canton, urban sector located on the road to Guayaquil, in front of the general cemetery of the canton, the Health Unit is a second level of health care, the service of our research is the sterilisation area of the General Hospital Dr. Liborio Panchana Sotomayor.

3.1.2. Duration of the proposed .

The proposal to be carried out has an implementation period of six months.

3.1.3. Background to the proposed .

The objective of occupational risks in the sterilisation area is to identify the risks that may occur with health personnel, to determine the negative effects caused by these risks, to draw up a plan of measures aimed at preventing them, and also to serve as a tool to unify prevention criteria.

The vast majority of accidents at work are avoidable, especially serious and fatal ones; accidents at work are not the consequence of a biblical curse or an unavoidable tribute of work, accidents are the result of the consequence of the lack of preventive practices which in their nature are knowable and applicable.

The General Hospital Dr. Liborio Panchana Sotomayor is the most complex unit of the health services network of the Province of Santa Elena, governed by policies and regulations dictated by the Ministry of Public Health of Ecuador, with continuous training,

It should be noted that such training should be prioritised to areas of higher occupational risk, such as the Central Sterilisation Unit, which has nine nurses.The sterilisation centre at the General Hospital of Santa Elena is considered to be the heart of the hospital. The occupational hazards that exist in the sterilisation area include all physical, mechanical, biological and preferably chemical procedures used to destroy pathogenic germs in which critical (instruments or objects that are introduced directly into the bloodstream, e.g. surgical instruments, implants, etc.) and semi-critical (which are in contact with the patient's intact mucous membranes, e.g. endotracheal tubes) manoeuvres are carried out, as the personnel run the risk of suffering intoxication, burns, eye irritation or irritation, as they are in contact with the patient's intact mucous membranes.These are in danger of poisoning, burns, eye irritation, lung problems, eyestrain, falls, allergies, cuts, fires, constant handling of contaminated material, lighting, noise, equipment failure, heat, electric shocks, sterilising gases, lifting of heavy instrumentation.

The personnel working in this area are not aware of the existence of an intervention plan to prevent accidents at work, because the administrative area has not paid attention to this area in order to have a highly trained and permanent staff, there are no signs to differentiate between contaminated and sterile areas, there is no frequent training for their knowledge, as they only work with auxiliary personnel and do not have professional staff in charge, where continuous supervision is carried out in order to make decisions prevent accidents at work in sterilisation centre.

In the sterilisation area, it is necessary to determine the negative effects that these risks have on health, and an intervention plan should be drawn up to prevent them, as well as tools that should be adopted to the safety standards and recommendations so that the personnel can obtain the corresponding protections.

It is part of all administrative management processes, supervisions and monitoring, quality indicators to carry out the analysis of existing hazards to avoid occupational risks to which the staff working in the sterilisation area of the General Hospital is exposed.

Dr. Liborio Panchana Sotomayor, as it does not have an Occupational Risk Intervention Plan.

3.1.4. Justification of the proposed .

In every health institution, the protection of human resources with regard to the risks in their working life must be guaranteed as a management measure according to the area of their development.We can determine which occupational hazards are the dangers existing in our work task or in our own environment or workplace, which can cause accidents or any type of accidents that, in turn, are factors that can cause injuries, physical or psychological damage, trauma, etc.

With this reference we consider implementing an intervention plan to avoid occupational risk in the sterilisation area of the General Hospital Dr. Liborio Panchana Sotomayor, Canton Santa Elena, Santa Elena province, as an alternative proposal for a solution.

In order to reduce occupational risk in sterilisation area in the population under study. The aim is to seek strategies to prevent accidents at work under an intervention plan that will benefit the overall health of employees.

3.1.5. Beneficiaries of the proposed .

Direct: Nurses from the sterilisation area of the Hospital Indirect: Health team of the health institution.

3.1.6. Feasibility technical feasibility.

The World Health Organisation states that the cornerstone of biosafety practice is risk assessment. Although many tools exist to help assess the risk involved in a given procedure or experiment, the most important component is professional judgement. Risk assessments should be carried out by those with the best knowledge of the specific characteristics of the organisms to be worked on, the equipment and the procedures to be used, with the aim of reducing the potential risks in the workplace. (WHO, 2023).

The research project has the characteristics, technical and operational conditions that ensure the fulfilment of its goals and objectives.

The process of a training programme complements the proposed actions and reinforces the components described to prevent accidents at work in the sterilisation area.

As an additional complement to the training, in order to multiply the beneficiaries, a prevention mechanism has been structured to avoid work-related accidents in the sterilisation area of General Hospital Dr. Liborio Panchana Sotomayor, Santa Elena Canton, Santa Elena Province.

The prevention of occupational risks is a priority in any work activity. In addition to being a legal, moral and social obligation of the employer, it requires the commitment and active participation of all members of the health institution.

The cornerstone of occupational safety practice is risk assessment, which should be carried out by persons who are most familiar with the characteristics of the institution, the equipment and the procedures to be used. Once the assessment has been completed, it should be reviewed periodically and whenever necessary, in order to prevent accidents at work in the sterilisation area.

3.1.7. Objectives of the proposed .

3.1.7.1. General objective of the proposed .

To avoid occupational hazards in the sterilisation area of the General Hospital Dr. Liborio Panchana Sotomayor, Santa Elena canton, Santa Elena Province.

3.1.7.2. Specific objectives of the proposed .

• Develop a design and systematisation of an intervention plan through training.
• Draw up an occupational health and risk prevention plan.

• Obtain a verification process under programming to avoid occupational hazards.

• Draw up a socialisation schedule for training in occupational risk and prevention measures.

3.1.8. LOGICAL FRAMEWORK MATRIX (Table N° 13)

LOGICAL FRAMEWORK				
	GOALS	INDICATOR	MEANS OF VERIFICATION	SUPPOSITIONS
FIN	To contribute to prevent occupational hazards in the sterilisation area of the General Hospital Dr. Liborio Panchana Sotomayor, Canton Santa Elena, Santa Elena Province.	Increase the knowledge of staff working in the sterilisation area to 75%.	Use of quality indicators	Personal decision for change
PURPOSE	Intervention Plan to avoid occupational risk in the sterilisation area the General Hospital Dr. Liborio Panchana Sotomayor, Santa Elena Canton, Santa Elena Province.	To reduce the number of occupational accidents by 75% among staff working in the sterilisation area.	Performance evaluation	Institutional reforms in the sector to be sustained, not catastrophes
COMPONENTS	Design and systematisation of an intervention plan through training. Occupational health and risk prevention plan: care protocols and application of management and quality indicators.	100% of the internal users (nurses) of the sterilisation centre applying the standardised procedures in the intervention plan.	Performance evaluation	Financial administrative processes
ACTIVITIES	Training of human talent in occupational hazards.			
	Training in occupational prevention measures Socialisation of user care protocols and application of management and quality indicators.			

Prepared by: Authors

3.1.9. Development of the proposed .

3.1.9.1. Design and systematisation of an intervention plan through training.

The design and systematisation of an intervention plan through training is important, since the General Hospital Dr. Liborio Panchana Sotomayor has a Teaching Unit within its structural organisation. Consequently, an intervention will be managed before the training and teaching department avoid occupational risks in the sterilisation area, with the aim of obtaining highly trained personnel in sterilisation processes, who are capable of integrating multidisciplinary teams, in order to guarantee:The microbiological quality of biomedical devices and instruments, suitable for their use and safety for the personnel who carry out sterilisation tasks, reducing occupational risks.

Training.

Training is a short-term educational process applied in a systematic and organised way,
through which people learn specific, work-related knowledge, attitudes towards aspects of the task organisation and environment and skills development.
The content of training can involve four types of behaviour change: Transmission of nformation.
Development and skills.
evelopment or modification of attitudes. Concept development.

Thus providing the theoretical and practical elements for health professionals and non-professionals to perform efficiently in their area of institutional work.
Its importance lies in the purpose of contributing with a basic tool for the personnel working in the sterilisation area, where it is necessary to comply with a high quality of knowledge in order to avoid occupational hazards, proposing a model of training and continuous development of learning to avoid occupational accidents in the sterilisation area.
It is intended that with the implementation of the design and systematisation of a training plan, the level of knowledge of nurses and other staff will be increased, improving the level of knowledge and thus increasing the prestige of the institution.

3.1.9.2. Occupational health and risk prevention plan.

In order for the sterilisation area to function properly, it is necessary for the personnel to be capable of observing the operating manuals and performance standards, which should establish in their contents from the basic principles to the most advanced and updated procedures.The objective is to provide the General Hospital Dr. Liborio Panchana Sotomayor with an instrument that serves as a guide to systematise the process of an occupational health and risk prevention plan and to strengthen professional development in the workplace. Occupational health and risk prevention plan is of great importance considering the application of a training and development model through the elaboration of specific action plans that carry a logical and timely sequence each of the phases of the training process.It involves the elaboration of a diagnosis of training and development needs related to the institution's occupational risks, the establishment of objectives, policies, programmes and a budget estimate in order to meet these needs and improve the level of staff performance.

Policies.

Institutions have policies that adequately lead to the achievement of the general objectives of the organisation or health institution, and it is also necessary to determine those that guide the training and development of the professional. These include the following:

Establish an ongoing training and development programme.

To take part in professional development of nursing through high quality training.

Actively include the areas involved in the teaching process for the prevention of occupational hazards.

Analyse the funding required for training where necessary.

Persistently assess whether the knowledge gained in training is being passed on to nurses and others.

Care protocols and application of management and quality indicators.

It should be emphasised that the sterilisation area is the most important operational part of the system or set of scientific procedures aimed at preserving equipment, instruments, materials, supplies or hospital facilities from germs or microbes, which should be considered as potentially infectious, and therefore sufficient precautions should be taken to prevent occupational hazards from occurring among healthcare personnel. The general objective is to systematise, advise, conduct and control the management of care and prevention of accidents at work, providing protocols and indicators of quality management in a comprehensive manner in the area of sterilisation at the different levels of surveillance with a focus on comprehensive primary health care, ensuring that this is of quality, warmth, timely and risk-free. An important part of quality management problems can be anticipated by taking action before they occur. This should be the approach favoured by the facility. The first step is to provide the health care institution with all the basic structural requirements that quality systems need to operate, and to implement evaluation processes in the different areas, especially in sterilisation, to avoid occupational hazards for the staff working there.

All the activities described in the sterilisation area of the hospital must have a person in charge and functions formally assigned by the institution. The assignment of roles and responsibilities may be included in the respective procedure manuals or protocols that regulate the activity, or may be included separately in independent documents determined by the institution.

Organisational structures should be put in place where reference should be made to the existence of specific organisational structures or models, e.g. a committee, or a centralised sterilisation system, should be written down in an institutional document. Verify that the structures have the necessary attributes, e.g. in terms of the profession or level of training of the members of the structure (in the case of the occupational risk control committee), or the functions to be performed. Assessment activities generally consist of systematic, periodic measurements of compliance with a practice in the sterilisation area, compared to a reference standard. The standard is the hospital's internal norm, protocol or institutional procedures manual, which indicates "how" these practices should be carried out.Compliance with the practice can be verified by review of records, computer records, supervisory activities or others. The results are most often expressed as a proportion of compliance with the standard (e.g. % of cases where the procedure was applied as intended in occupational accident prevention). Other variants of evaluation activities include audits against adverse events, surveys and evaluations of a qualitative nature. In general we can analyse that quality indicators can be defined as "measurable parameters, explicitly defined, which refer to structures, processes or results of care, and which are judged to be linked to the quality of care". Their main objectives are: to document the quality of processes in the sterilisation area, and to evaluate their trend, to document results, and to compare them with reference standards or to evaluate their trend in order to avoid occupational hazards.

3.1.9.3. Verification process under programming to avoid occupational hazards.

The general purpose is to boost the efficiency of the sterilisation centre, training to contribute to raising the level of knowledge and therefore the efficiency of human talent in the prevention of accidents at work and to improve the integration of work teams.
Lack of knowledge refers to the lack of awareness of the existence of the recommendation given by the institution. Many health professionals simply do not apply procedures because they are unaware that an institutional standard, protocol or manual exists, or because they have not taken the time to review it.
At the end of a training and development event, the level of learning of the nursing staff and other participants must be verified in order to provide feedback on their knowledge and evaluate their performance, using evaluation instruments, as well as obtaining information related to the cost-benefit of the training and recording the attendance of staff in training. It is essential to follow up the training by carrying out actions to verify that the knowledge acquired is put into practice with the general objective of preventing occupational hazards in the sterilisation area of the institution.

3.1.9.4. Socialisation schedule for training in occupational risk and prevention measures.

A training plan to prevent occupational hazards in the sterilisation area should be socialised and disseminated to raise awareness among health personnel (nurses), as well as users and external beneficiaries. In view of the above, information and training should be provided on labour rights and obligations, occupational diseases and biological risks that may occur in the sterilisation area, and basic principles of action should be established to prevent risks of accidents and occupational diseases, to protect the health of health personnel, and to place and maintain them in an occupation in accordance with their physiological and psychological conditions.Regularly implement continuous training programmes for the protection of the internal users of the sterilisation area. It is worth noting that the health team working in a second level of care hospital establishment is exposed to innumerable risks, capable of causing alterations or occupational pathologies, and sterilisation services are no exception for the occurrence of occupational risks. On the contrary, we can state that it constitutes a workplace that entails a high occupational risk, which can be of a different nature, the most common being: physical, chemical, biological and ergonomic.Training, communication and internal regulation as primary strategies to prevent occupational hazards, and the application of physical and chemical barrier activities, proper waste management and its universality, maintaining a direct relationship with the health team to quickly identify environmental factors (humidity, steam, heat), which affect the normal limits of comfort. Train staff on proper working postures and the natural movements to be applied when moving loads, lifting weights, etc. Bearing in mind the use of aids such as mobilisation or appropriate mechanical equipment, to avoid fatigue and musculoskeletal disorders. Establish a rotation of activities among staff to avoid work monotony. The plan also includes the risk assessment, protective measures, emergency plan as well as updating measures. In order to prevent occupational hazards, the sterilisation area must comply with the applicable regulations of the occupational risk management. Direct supervision of the unit, with physical presence of the unit by experts in field, carrying out direct control of the sterilisation area, in terms of hygiene and safety of the health team working in the sterilisation area. The main objective is to have management policies to avoid occupational risks in the sterilisation area, in order to incorporate a preventive attitude on the part of the nursing staff working in the hospital, continuously developing intervention plans under programming and effective socialisation.

3.1.9.5. Timetable for the implementation of the proposal (Table N° 13)

ACTIVITIES	YEAR 2015						RESPONSIBLE
	APRIL	MAY	JUNE	JULY	AUGUST	SEPTEMBER	
Designing and systematising a training intervention plan							Director of the General Hospital Dr. Liborio Panchana Sotomayor
Occupational health and risk prevention plan: care protocols and application of management and quality indicators.							
Socialisation schedule for training in occupational risk and prevention .							
Verification: programming to avoid occupational hazards.							
Prepared by: Authors							

3.1.9.6. Intervention Plan Table 14)

Knowledge of occupational hazards among nursing staff working in the sterilisation area of the General Hospital Dr. Liborio Panchana Sotomayor.

Objective: To contribute to the improvement of the working environment of the nursing staff in the sterilisation area of the H.G.L.P.S., raising awareness and sensitising the authorities and staff to these issues and how to reduce and/or prevent them.

PROBLEM	ACTIONS	RESPONSIBLE	TIME	OBSERVATION
Insufficient knowledge of institutional authorities and nursing staff regarding occupational hazards.	Transfer of the research document prepared in order to raise awareness among the authorities and senior management of the occupational hazards to which nursing staff are exposed in the area of sterilisation.	Hospital authorities	20 hours	Seminar-workshop
	Design and implement a training plan on occupational hazards in the sterilisation area. Carry out a training and awareness-raising plan on occupational hazards in the sterilisation area.			
High rate of ergonomic, physical and psychosocial occupational hazards.	Design and implement procedural standards for ergonomic, physical and psychosocial occupational hazards. Universal precautions Use of protective elements.	Director/Manager of the Institution		
Prepared by: Authors				

3.1.9.7. Educational training event on occupational hazards for nursing staff working in the sterilisation area of the General Hospital Dr. Liborio Panchana Sotomayor (Table N° 15).

Competence: To develop in the nursing staff knowledge and skills that allow them to orientate with a theoretical-practical instrument in front of the different risks that are generated in the sterilization area of the H.G.L.P.S. **Hours:** 20 hours

SPECIFIC COMPETENCES	ISSUES	METHODOLOGY	EVALUATION CRITERION	LOGISTICAL SUPPORT
Critical and analytical tendency in the application of rules and procedures for the prevention of occupational hazards.	Risk Definition Fundamentals of occupational health and safety Health Illness Relationship between health and work. Risks: Biological Chemical Chemical Ergonomic Physical Physical Psychosocial. Accident, occupational disease, legal regulations	Development: Welcome Knowledge assessment. Didactic presentation by the speaker with the support of the nursing staff, Question and answer session to clarify participants' doubts. Final: Group workshop Problem-based learning	Applies safe working procedures: 1.-Precautions model 2.- Handling of sharp and hot material 3.- Proper fitting and use of personal protective equipment. Correct application of procedures in case of accidents.	Events room. Image projector. Acrylic blackboard. Annotation sheet. Pencils. Markers.
Prepared by: Authors				

3.1.9.8. Total budget (Table N° 16)

PROPOSAL	YEAR 2024
Design and systematisation of a training plan.	$ 700,00
Occupational health and risk prevention plan: care protocols and application of management and quality indicators.	$ 870,00
Socialisation schedule for training in occupational risk and prevention measures.	$ 50,00
Verification: programming to avoid occupational hazards.	$ 50,00
Coffee break.	$ 150,00
TOTAL:	$ 1.820,00
Prepared by: Authors	

3.2. VALIDATION OF THE PROPOSAL.

Dr. Manuel San Martín Abarca, with technical skills in administrative and hospital care management and primary health care, has been considered as the expert research structure for the validation of the proposal, which is viable and feasible.

3.3. Partial conclusions of the chapter.

After proposing an intervention plan to prevent occupational hazards in the sterilisation area, the following conclusions were reached:The objective of occupational risks in the sterilisation area is to identify the risks that may occur with health personnel, to determine the negative effects caused by these risks, to draw up a plan of measures aimed at preventing them, and also to serve as a tool to unify prevention criteria. The general objective is to avoid occupational hazards in the sterilisation area of the General Hospital Dr. Liborio Panchana Sotomayor, Santa Elena, Santa Elena Province. The purpose of the intervention plan is to prevent occupational hazards in the sterilisation area of the General Hospital Dr. Liborio Panchana Sotomayor, Canton Santa Elena, Santa Elena Province, and to contribute to preventing occupational hazards in the sterilisation area of the General Hospital Dr. Liborio Panchana Sotomayor, Canton Santa Elena, Santa Elena Province.The following components were used: Design and systematisation of an intervention plan by means of training, 2. Plan for occupational health and risk prevention, 3. The following activities were carried out: Training of human talent in occupational hazards, training in occupational prevention measures and application of management and quality indicators.

GENERAL CONCLUSIONS.

Once the sterilisation area of the General Hospital Dr. Liborio Panchana Sotomayor has been investigated, in accordance with the lines of investigation and following the indications of the current research manual, we can conclude that:Through the investigation carried out, it was possible to identify that the nursing staff are providing care without knowledge in the management of the sterilisation area in order to avoid preventable accidents at work, due to inexperience due to lack of training in the updating of risk knowledge.The nursing staff is unaware of and has weaknesses in the identification of factors, as well as the non-use of fundamental strategies, due to the lack of training to act in the sterilisation area, all these factors have caused them to avoid occupational hazards in the hospital.The lack of an intervention plan to manage occupational risk strategies to prevent accidents has directly affected the wellbeing of the staff working in the sterilisation area and therefore has an impact on the preventive health of all the institution's staff.

RECOMMENDATIONS

Following the general conclusions of the research it is recommended that:
• To the health institution to study and accept the proposal of an intervention plan to avoid occupational risks in the sterilisation area, considering the basic strategies of prevention, promotion and socialisation of occupational accidents, in compliance with the objectives set out.
• At management level, conduct regular analysis and monitoring of occupational risks timely decision-making to ensure the integrity of the health team.
• Training for the entire health team on the importance of avoiding occupational hazards and their impact on the physical integrity of health personnel.
• An intervention plan should be socialised and disseminated through training to prevent occupational risks in the sterilisation area in order to raise awareness among health personnel (nurses), as well as users and external beneficiaries.

BIBLIOGRAPHY

Aguilar, E. (2021). Proceso de control y Mejoramiento de Salud Pública. Quito, Ecuador.
Ambriz Tapia, A. (2018). The Intervention Project. Intervention Projects.

Diploma in Urban Management.
Benenson, A. (2006). Manual for the Control of Communicable Diseases in Man.
Washington: Scientific Publication No. 564.

Castro, S. A. (2017). Peripheral Unit for the Prevention of Occupational Risks. Spain.
Andean Community, C. (2005). Resolution 957 Reglamento del instrumento Andino de
seguridad y salud en el trabajo.

Constituent, A. (2008). Constitution of the Republic of Ecuador. Alfaro.
Cortes, J. (2007). Tecnicas de prevencion de riesgos laborales, seguridad e higiene en el
trabajo. Madrid, Spain: Tébar.

School of Biomedical Engineering, E. S. (2017). Hospital Safety Manual. Faculty of Medical
Sciences, U. d. (2021).
Ferlie, E. (2017). The new public management in action. Oxford: Oxford University Press.
Fernandez, S. (2012). Bajas Coberturas. La Tercera.
Fierro, M. (2021). Risk factors in the Hospital Sterilisation Centre.

Latacunga.
Fuster Ruiz, M. (2008). Design of intervention projects. Mexico. Ignacio, U. S. (2020).
Classification of Occupational Risks. Bogotá.
MAIS-FCI 2018. (n.d.). Manual del Modelo de Atención Integral de Salud, Familiar,
Comunitario e Intercultural. Quito Ecuador.

Ministry of Public Health, C. (2020).

Ministry of Public Health, E. (2022). Manual de Normas Técnicos - Administrativos. Quito.
Molina, G. (2009). Trends in health services management. National School of Public Health,
73.

MOH (2022). Management of infectious waste in the health services network of Ecuador.
Quito.

NATURA, F. (2003). Seguridad y Salud Ocupacional. Quito.
NIOSH. (2007). Occupational Hazards in Sterilisation. Publication No. 2000-108. WHO.
(2023). Biosafety manual (3rd edition). Mexico.
OPS. (2022). Health and Safety of Health Sector Workers. Washington, DC.
Patón Jesús, M. (2021). Guia Básica de riesgos laborales específicos en el sector sanitario.
Health Federation and sectors.
Patón, J. M. (2021). Guia básica de riesgos Laborales.
Rodriguez, M. (2015). Central de Esterilización. Havana Cuba.
Román, A. (2012). Basic concepts and definitions of clinical management. Biomedical
Journal.

Ruiz, C. (2010). World Health Organization/Pan American Health Organization. Public Health, M. (2018). Manual de Normas y Procedimientos. Quito.

Velasco, L. (2018). Pracicas Preventivas. Quito.

ANNEXES

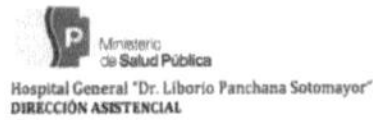

Ministerio
de Salud Pública

Hospital General "Dr. Liborio Panchana Sotomayor"
DIRECCIÓN ASISTENCIAL

Santa Elena, 04 de febrero del 2015

CERTIFICADO

QUE EL SUSCRITO DIRECTOR MÉDICO ASISTENCIAL DEL HOSPITAL GENERAL "DR. LIBORIO PANCHANA SOTOMAYOR" CERTIFICA:

Que la señorita licenciada **SAAVEDRA ALVARADO ELSIE ANTONIETA** con C.I. 1204481608 realizó como estructura de trabajo de investigación, previo a la obtención del título de Magíster en Gerencia de Servicios de Salud de la Universidad Regional Autónoma de los Andes, extensión Santo Domingo, con el tema: **PLAN DE INTERVENCIÓN PARA EVITAR EL RIESGO LABORAL EN EL ÁREA DE ESTERILIZACIÓN EN EL HOSPITAL GENERAL "DR. LIBORIO PANCHANA SOTOMAYOR, CANTÓN SANTA ELENA, PROVINCIA SANTA ELENA.**

La misma que doy fe a la validación de la propuesta siendo esta viable y factible para la Institución de Salud.

Autorizo a la interesada a hacer uso del que estime conveniente al presente documento.

Es todo lo que puede certificar en honor a la verdad.

Atentamente,

Dr. Miguel San Martín Abarca
DIRECTOR MÉDICO ASISTENCIAL HGLPS
C.c.   Archivo.-

		SUMILLA
ELABORADO:	Ninfa Rengifo M.	
REVISADO:	Dr. Miguel San Martín	
APROBADO:	Abarca	

Av. Marquez de la Plata S/N frente al Cementerio de Santa Elena
Teléfonos: 593 (4) 2942611 ext: 171
www.msp.gob.ec

ANNEX # 1. QUESTIONNAIRE OF QUESTIONS FOR THE SURVEY OF STERILISATION AREA NURSING STAFF HOSPITAL GENERAL DR. LIBORIO PANCHANA SOTOMAYOR SANTA ELENA GENERAL HOSPITAL REGIONAL AUTONOMOUS UNIVERSITY OF THE ANDES SANTO DOMINGO EXTENSION POSTGRADUATE UNIT MASTER'S DEGREE IN HEALTH SERVICES MANAGEMENT

SELECT THE CORRECT BOX WITH AN X

1. *Knowledge of a Manual of Procedures-Protocols for the prevention of occupational risks in sterilisation? for the prevention of occupational risks in sterilisation?*
Yes No

2. *Does the hospital unit have a sterilisation quality and occupational risk prevention committee?*
Yes No

3. *Identification of occupational risk factors in the sterilisation area?*

Chemicals Ergonomic Physical Physical Biological Psychosocial

4. *Are systems or circulation routes in the sterilisation area well lit?*
Yes No

5. *Are materials and means of protection available to protect against accidents in the sterilisation area?*
Yes No

6. *Regular removal of stains or residues of hazardous substances or contaminants in the sterilisation area?*
Yes No

7. *Accidents with short sharp material cuts and/or punctures?*
Yes No

8. *Training on the handling of sterilisation equipment and its ?*
Yes No

9. *Knowledge of the nursing staff's instructions for action in an accident with biological, chemical or other material?*
Yes No

10. *Existence of conflicts between nursing staff in the sterilisation area?*

Yes No

11. *Does the hospital unit have an intervention plan to prevent occupational hazards in the sterilisation area?*
Yes No
Prepared by: *Authors*

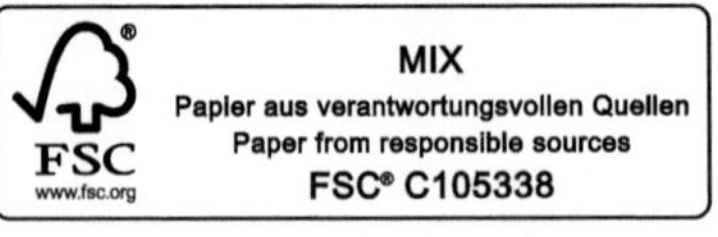

MIX
Papier aus verantwortungsvollen Quellen
Paper from responsible sources
FSC® C105338
FSC
www.fsc.org